UPDOG

DEADLY DISEASES

SMALLPOX

A Vaccine Success

Brianna Kaiser

Lerner Publications ◆ Minneapolis

Lerner Publications Company
An imprint of Lerner Publishing Group, Inc.
241 First Avenue North
Minneapolis, MN 55401 USA

For reading levels and more information, look up this title at www.lernerbooks.com.

Main body text set in ITC Franklin Gothic Std.
Typeface provided by Adobe Systems.

Designer: Mary Ross
Lerner team: Sue Marquis

Library of Congress Cataloging-in-Publication Data

Names: Kaiser, Brianna, 1996– author.
Title: Smallpox : a vaccine success / Brianna Kaiser.
Description: Minneapolis : Lerner Publications, [2022] | Series: Deadly diseases (updog books) | Includes bibliographical references and index. | Audience: Ages 8–11 | Audience: Grades 4–6 | Summary: “Scientists won the battle against smallpox. Young readers will learn all about the worldwide initiative to eradicate the disease and its final outbreak”—Provided by publisher.
Identifiers: LCCN 2020043808 (print) | LCCN 2020043809 (ebook) | ISBN 9781728428376 (library binding) | ISBN 9781728431260 (paperback) | ISBN 9781728430645 (ebook)
Subjects: LCSH: Smallpox—Juvenile literature. | Smallpox—Prevention—Juvenile literature.
Classification: LCC RC183 .K35 2022 (print) | LCC RC183 (ebook) | DDC 616.9/12—dc23

LC record available at https://lccn.loc.gov/2020043808
LC ebook record available at https://lccn.loc.gov/2020043809

Manufactured in the United States of America
1-49374-49478-2/25/2021

Table of Contents

Smallpox

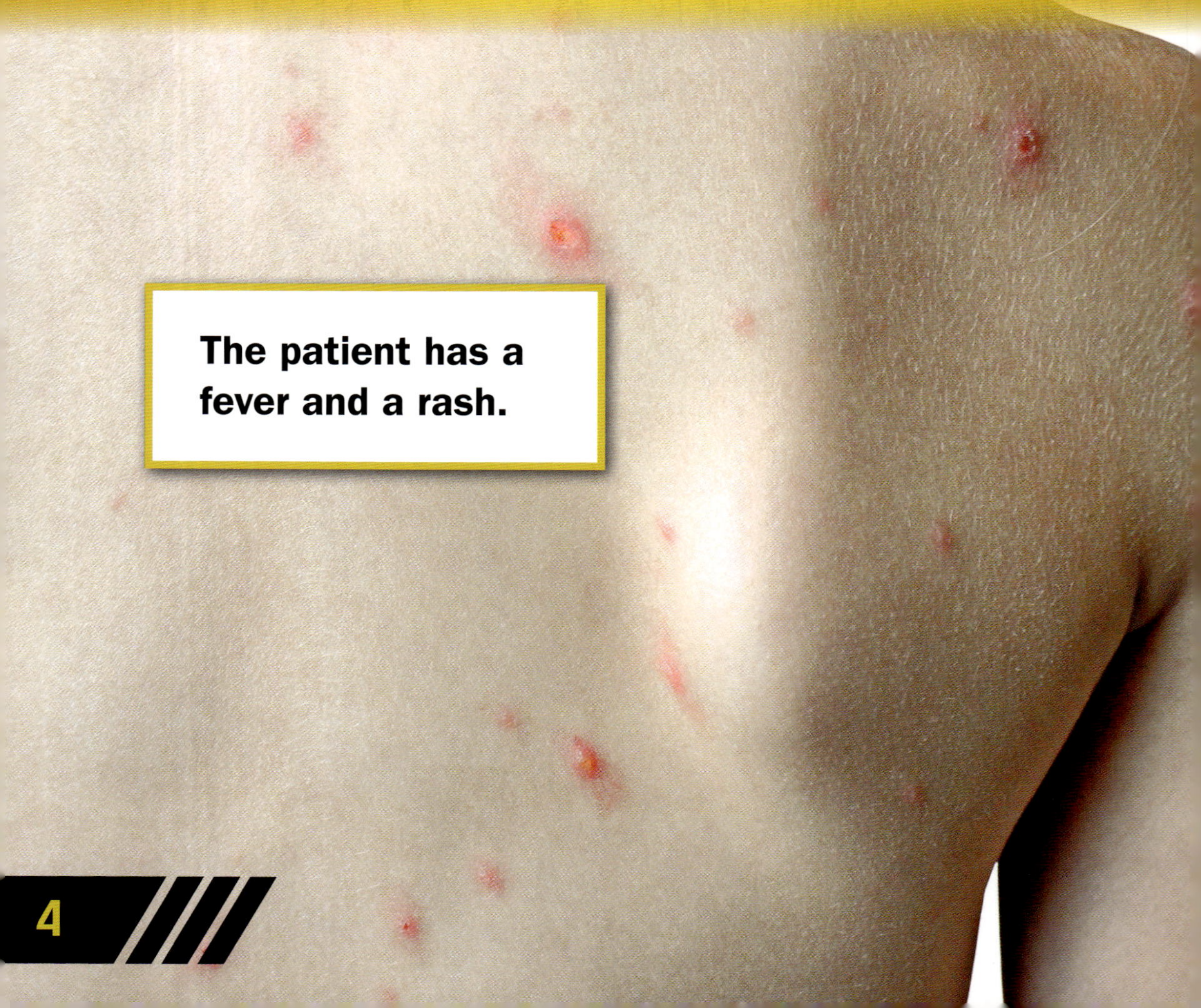

The patient has a fever and a rash.

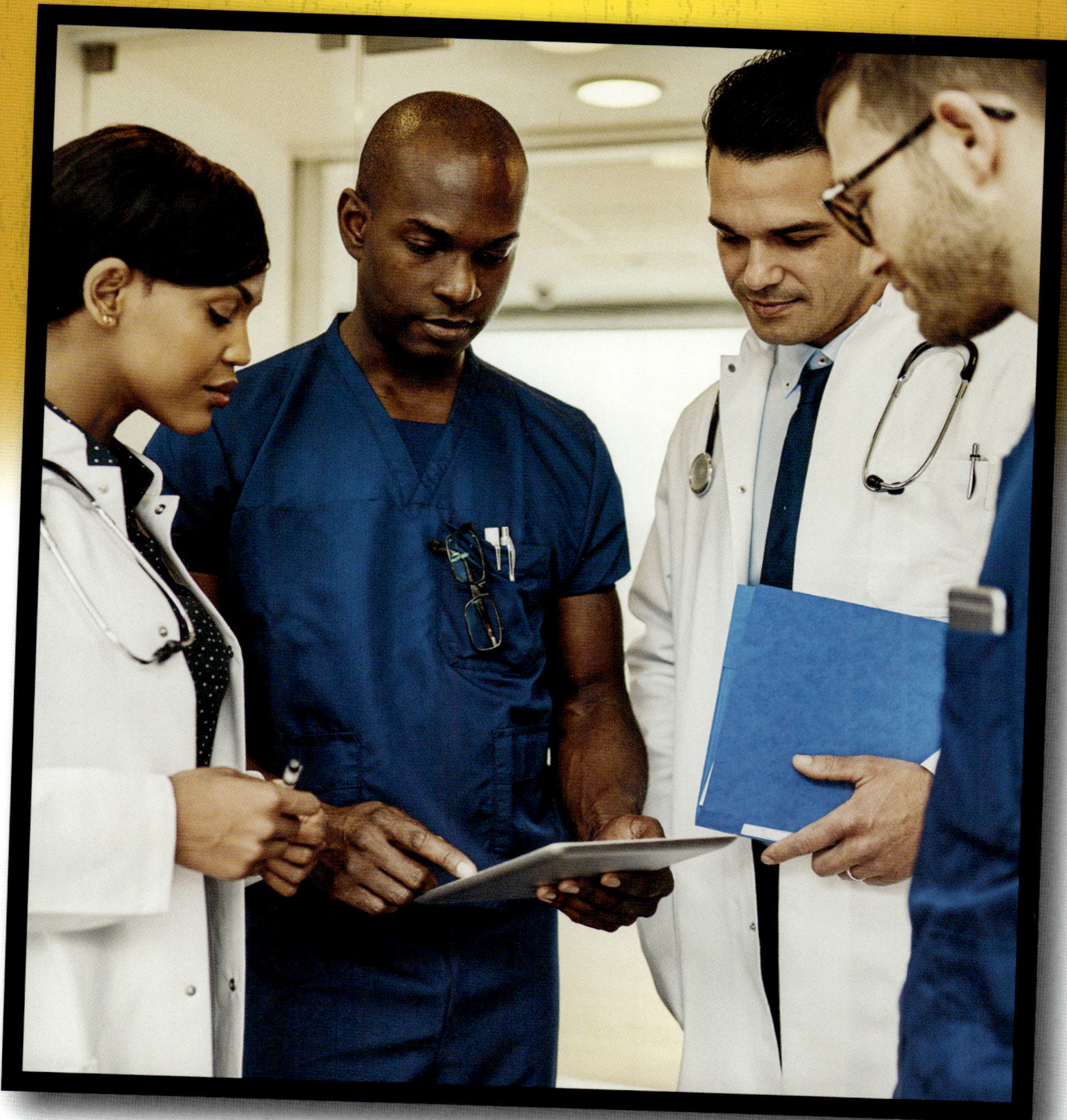

Doctors say it's smallpox.

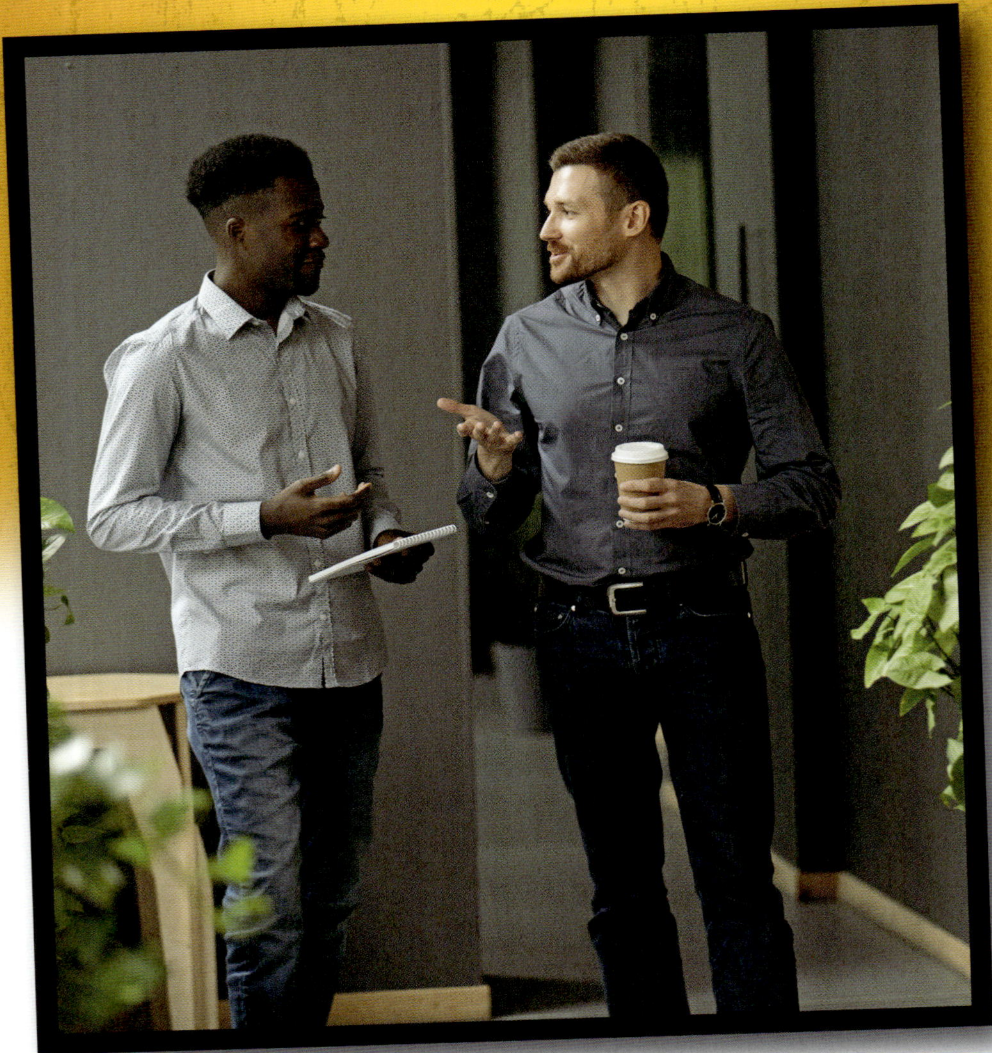

Smallpox is caused by a virus. It spreads from person to person.

virus: something that causes disease

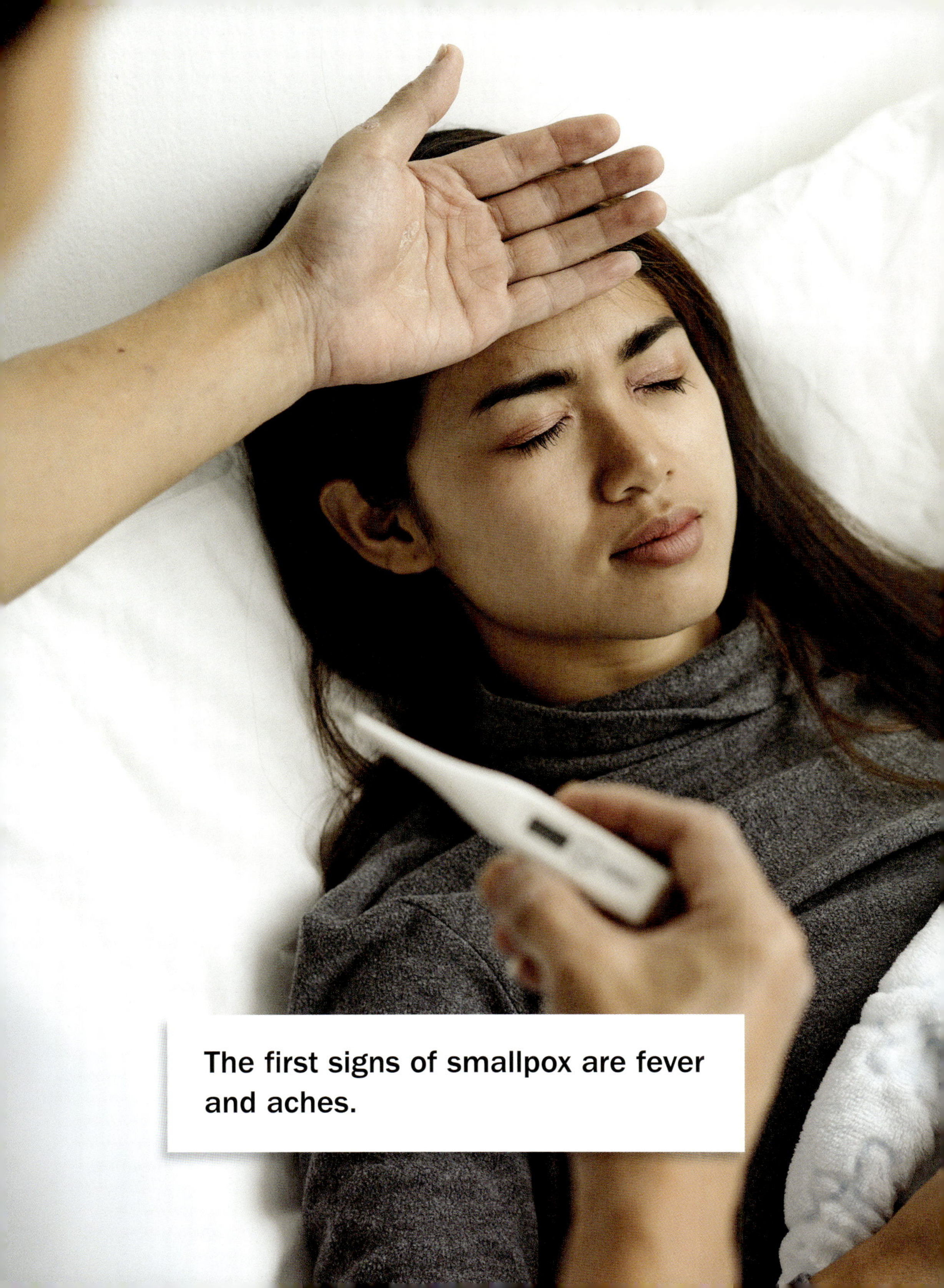

The first signs of smallpox are fever and aches.

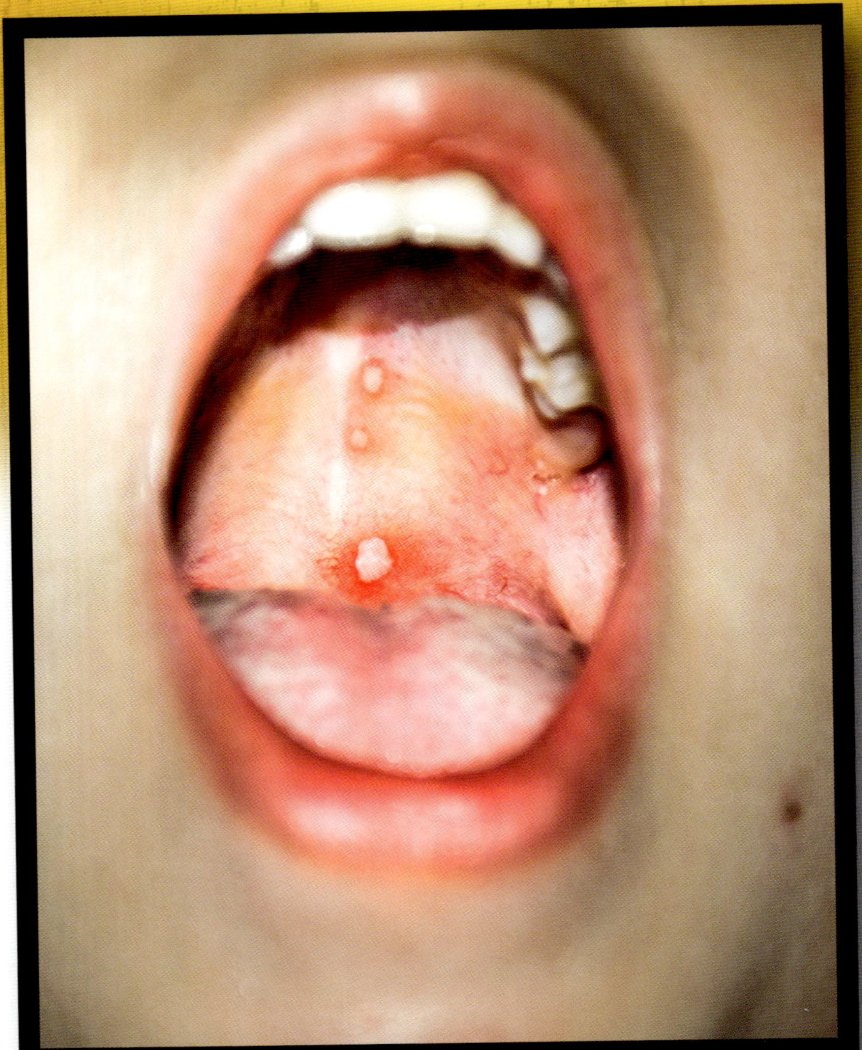

A few days later, small spots appear on the tongue and mouth.

Then a rash spreads across the body. The rash starts to scab. When all the scabs fall off, the person feels better.

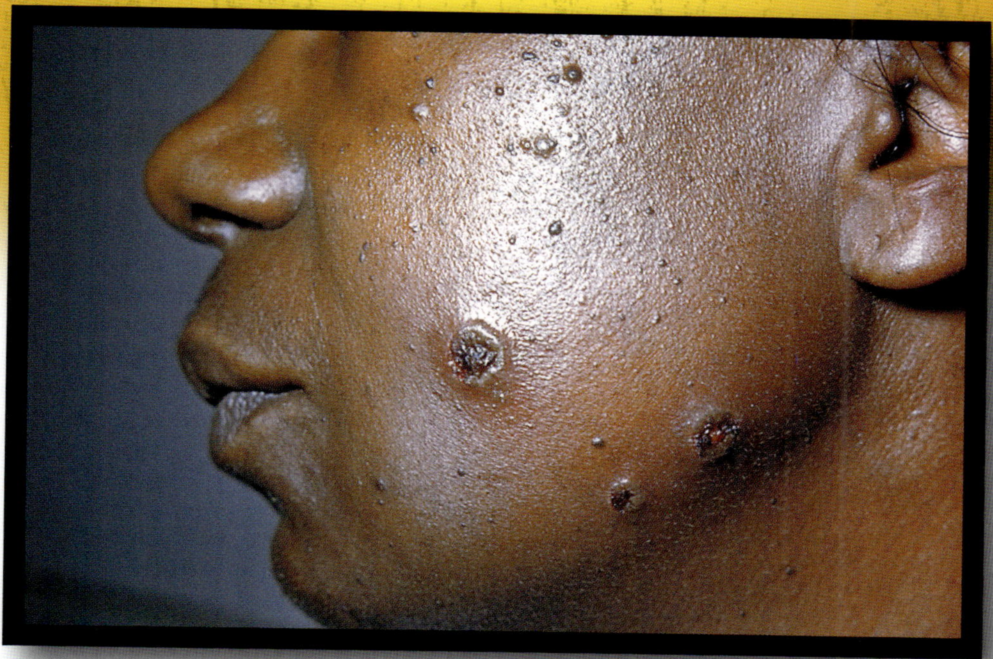

UP NEXT!
The Disease's Past.

The History of Smallpox

Smallpox is ancient. Travelers spread it around the world.

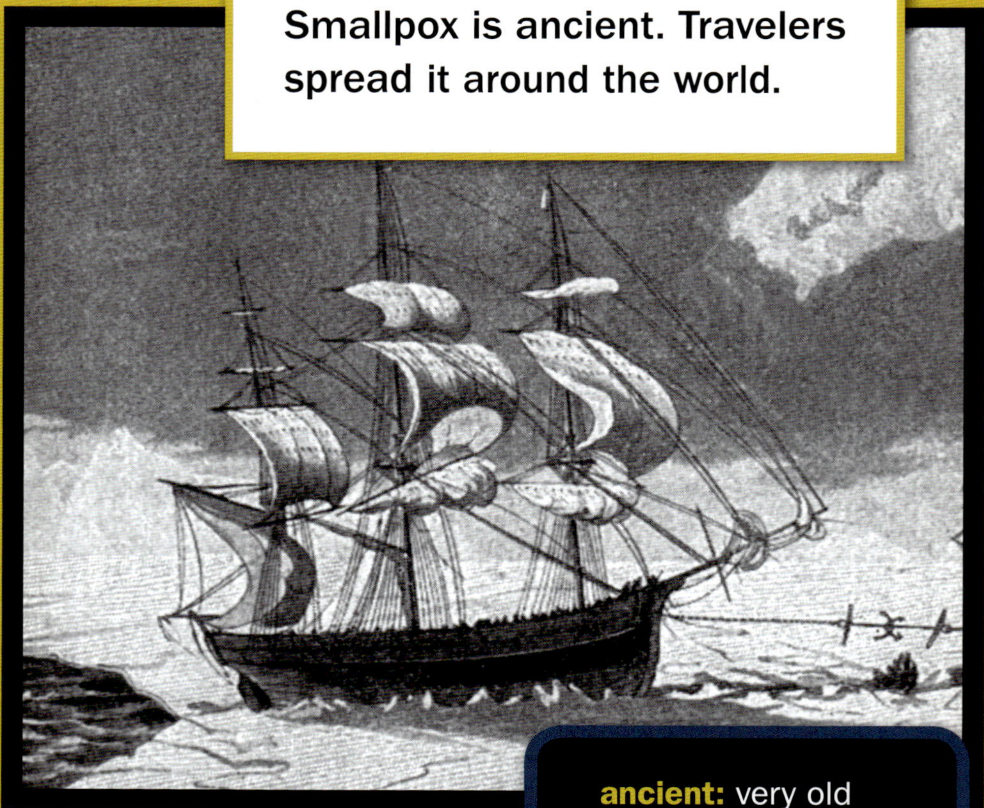

ancient: very old

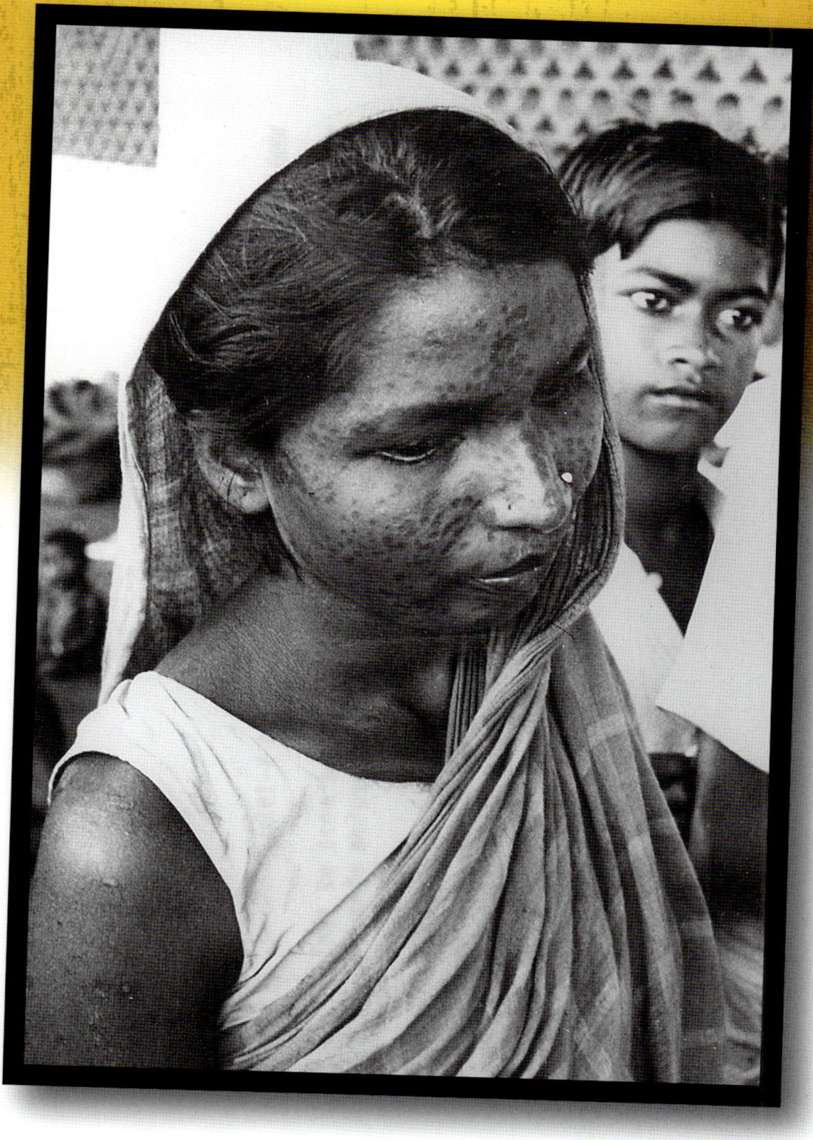

It gave some people scars. Many others died.

UP CLOSE

The image on the right shows the smallpox virus.

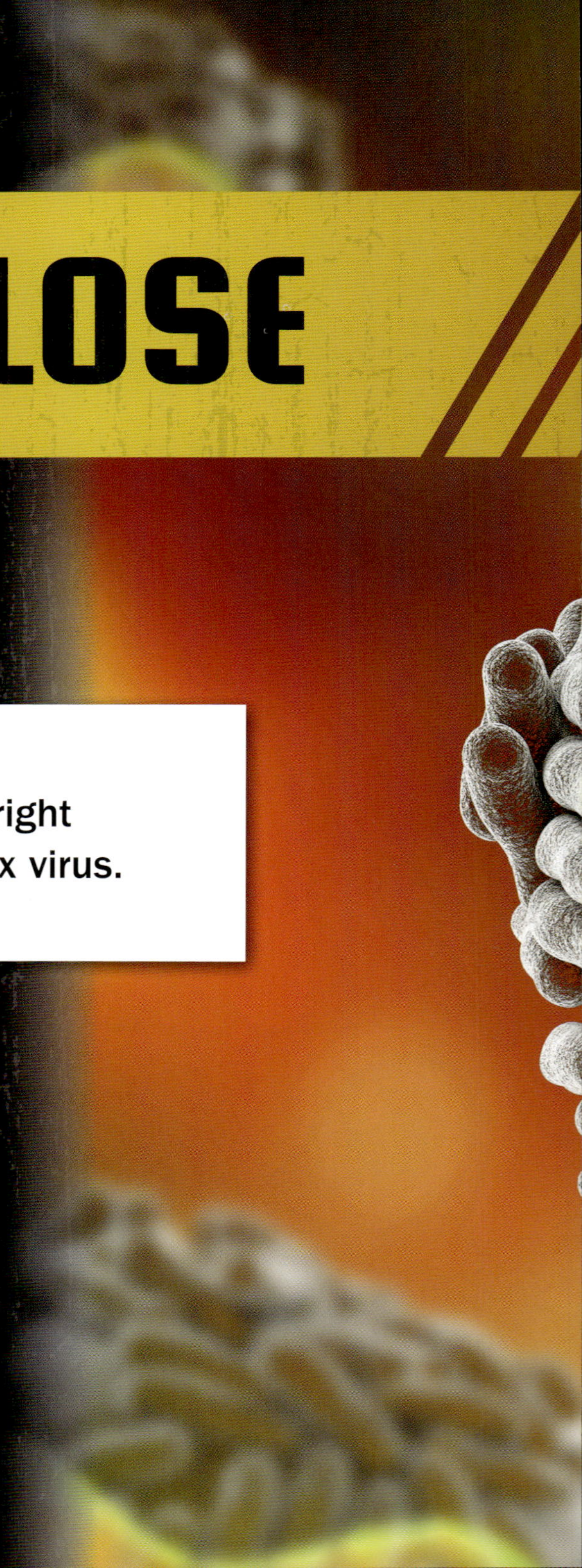

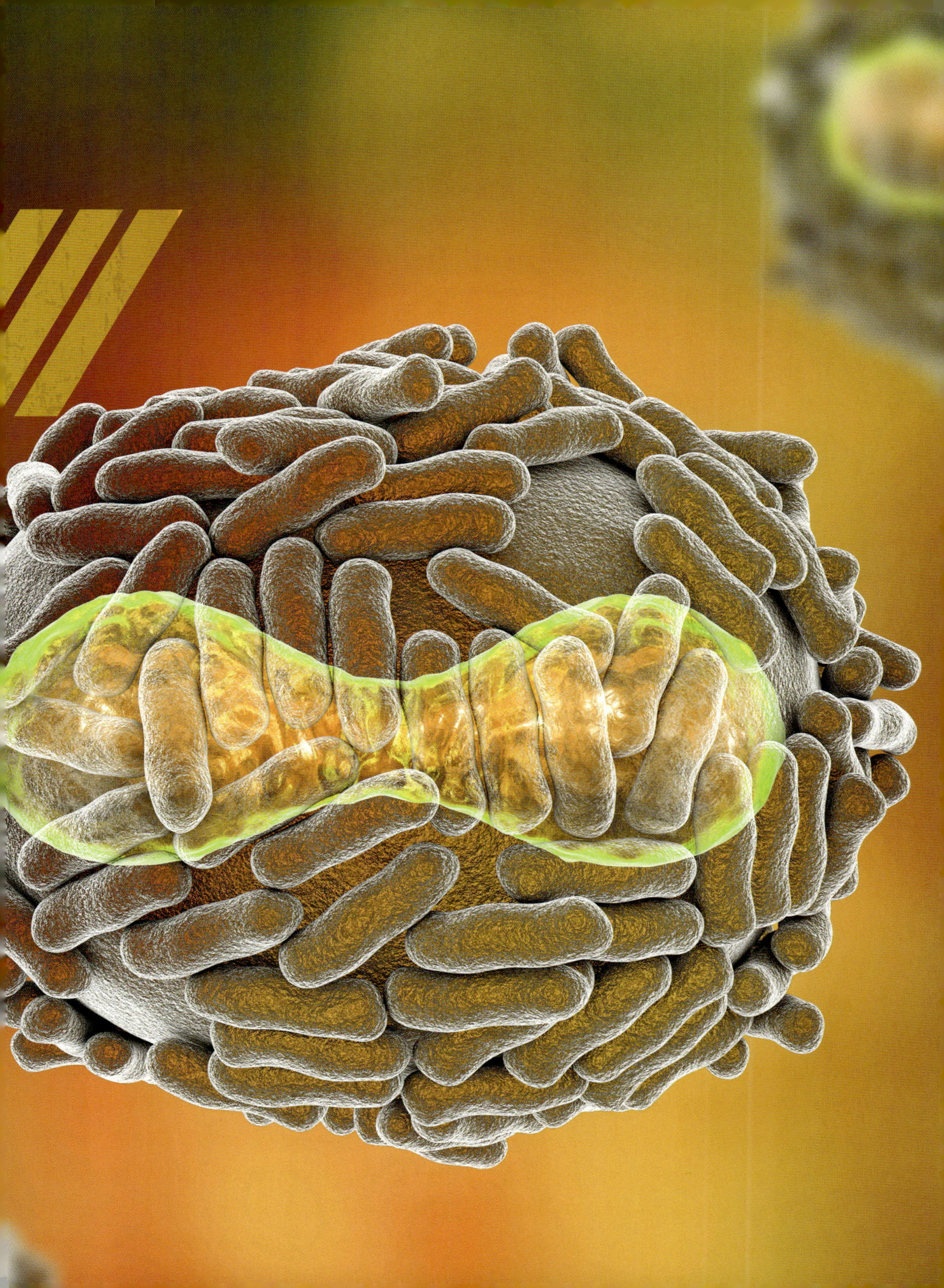

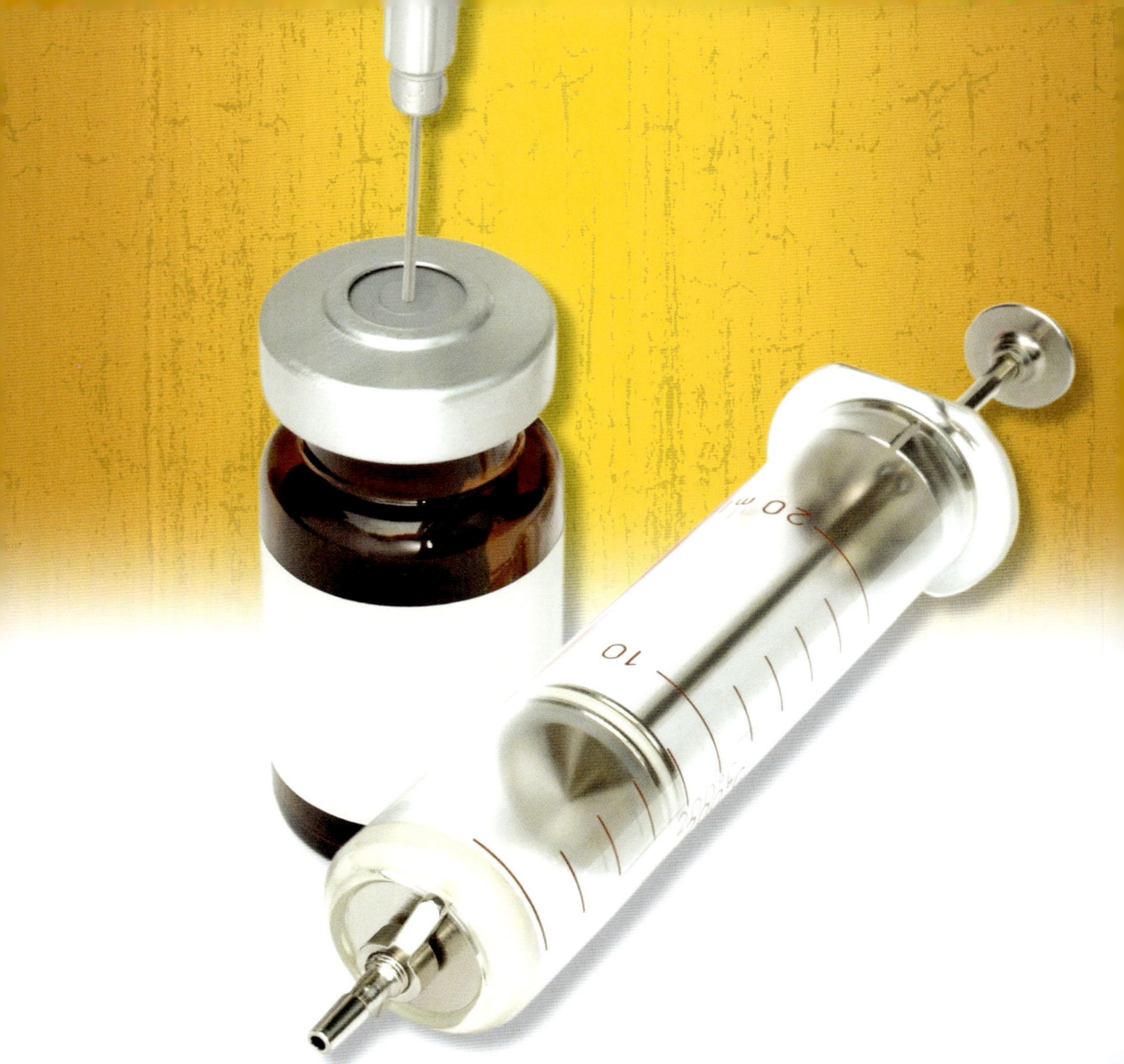

The first smallpox vaccine was used in the late 1700s.

vaccine: a shot to prevent disease

It helped keep people from getting sick.

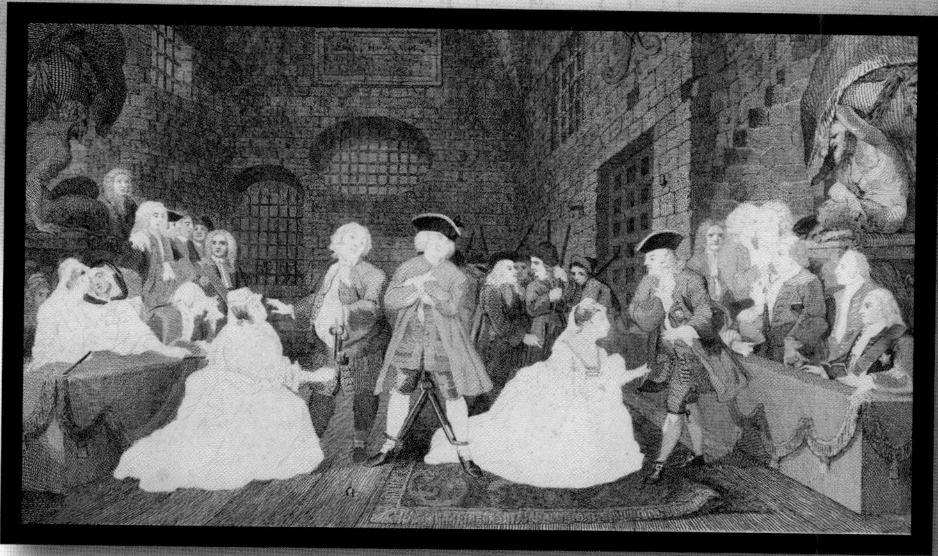

UP NEXT!
Stopping the Disease.

Stopping Smallpox

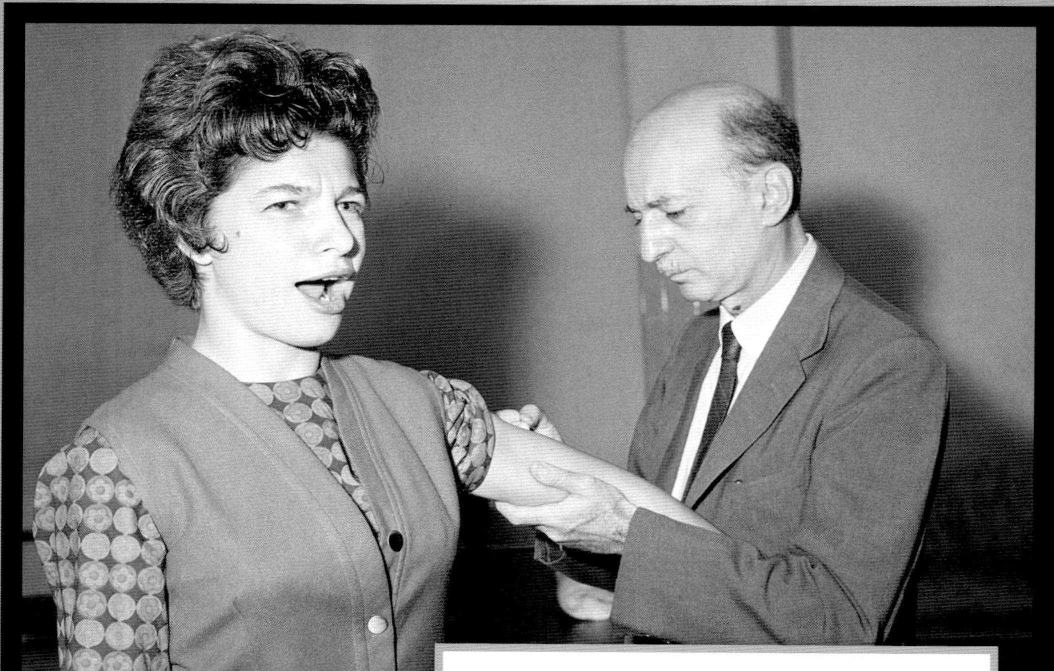

In 1967, doctors started a program to stop smallpox's spread.

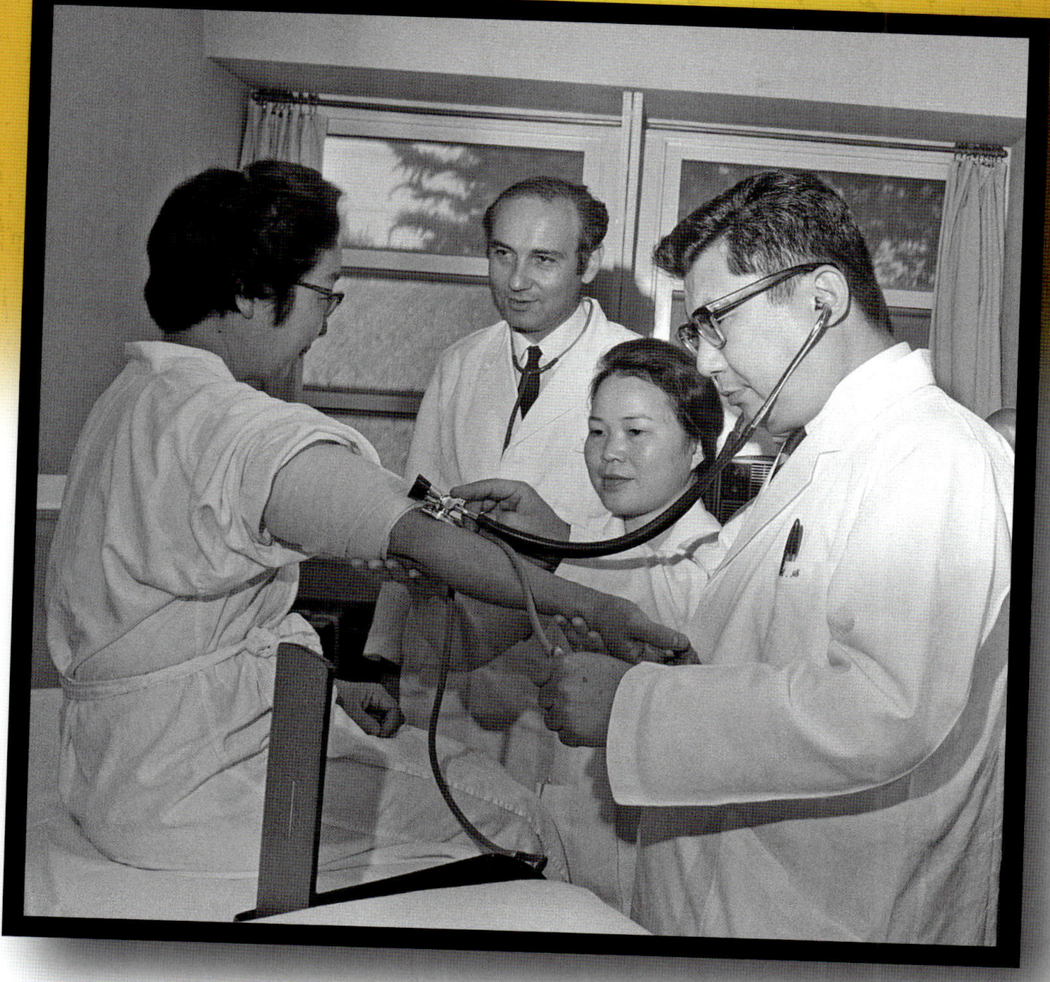

The last known case was in 1977.

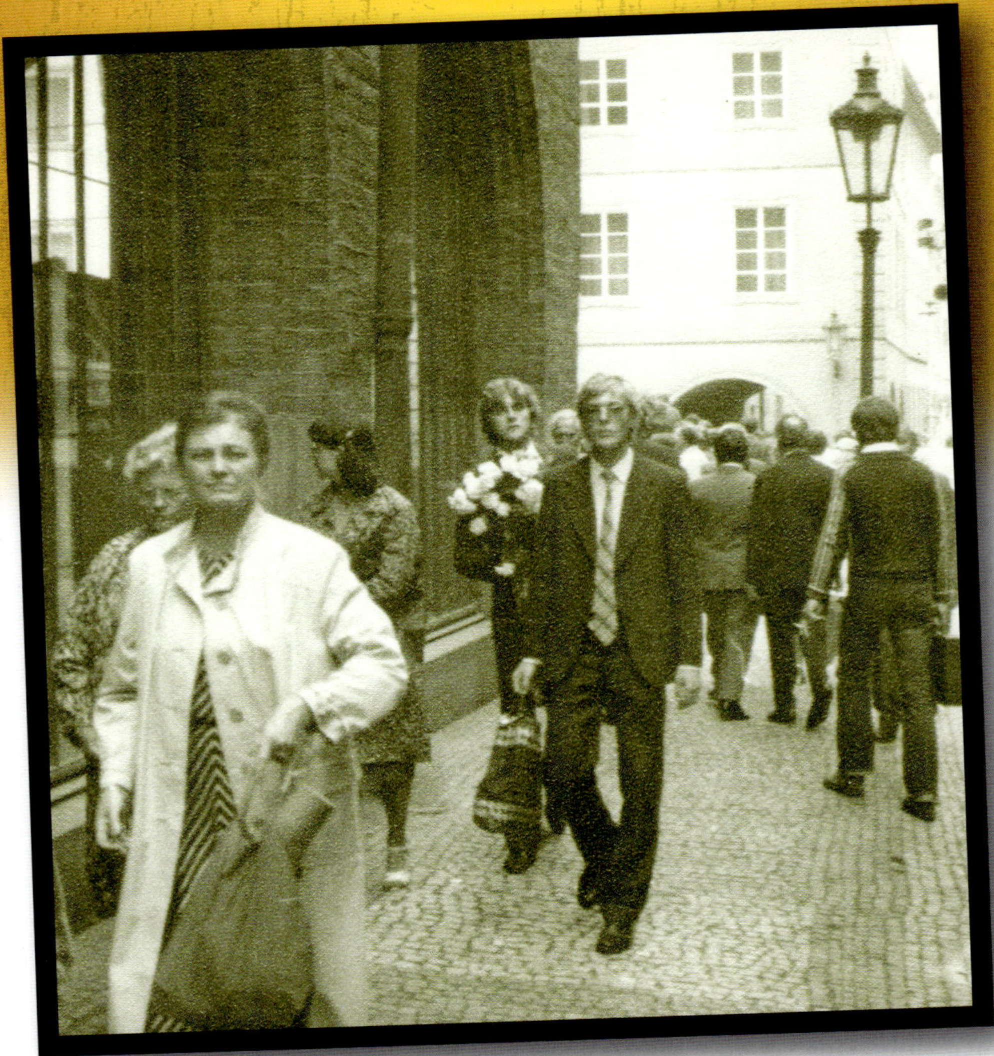

By 1980, the world was officially free of it.

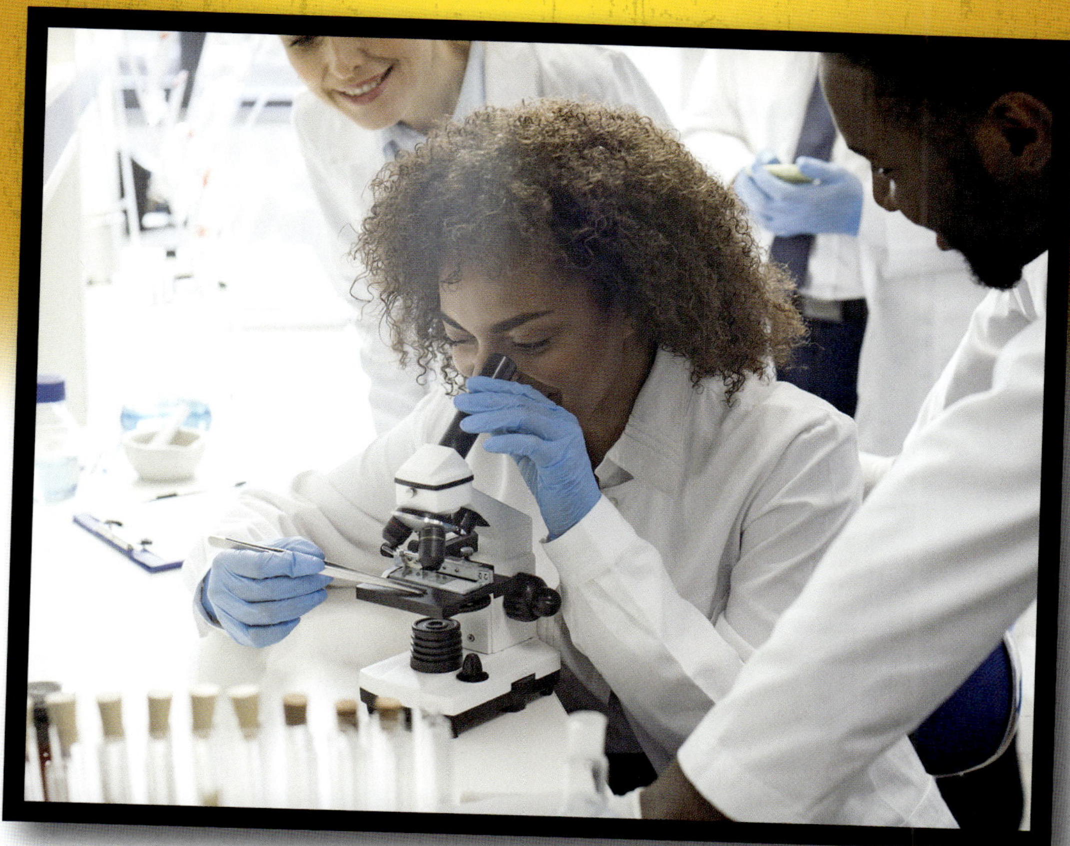

Scientists still research smallpox.

They want to be ready if it returns.

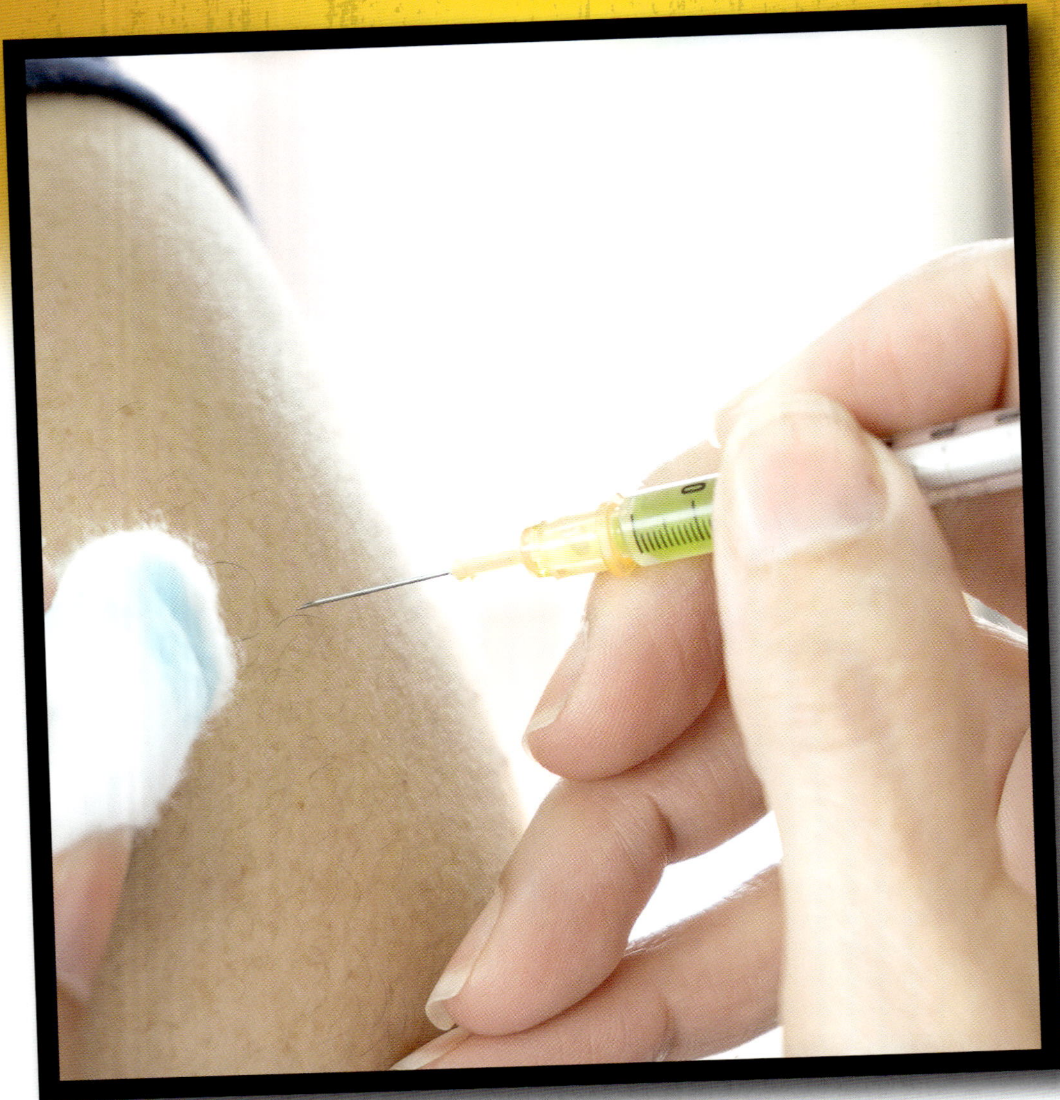

DOCTOR YOU!

Which patient do you think has smallpox?

Patient A	Patient B
fever	fever
cough	rash
aches	aches

Answer: Patient B

Glossary

ancient: very old

vaccine: a shot to prevent disease

virus: something that causes disease

Check It Out!

Kaiser, Brianna. *Malaria: An Ongoing Threat.* Minneapolis: Lerner Publications, 2022.

Leed, Percy. *Skin and Hair (A Sickening Augmented Reality Experience)*. Minneapolis: Lerner Publications, 2021.

Mould, Steve. *The Bacteria Book*. New York: DK, 2018.

Smallpox
https://kids.britannica.com/kids/article/smallpox/399600

Smallpox Facts for Kids
https://kids.kiddle.co/Smallpox

What Are Germs?
https://kidshealth.org/en/kids/germs.html

Index

Photo Acknowledgments

Image credits: Meryll/Shutterstock.com, p. 4; Flamingo Images/Shutterstock.com, p. 5; fizkes/Shutterstock.com, p. 6; Pormezz/Shutterstock.com, p. 7; Moon Safari/Shutterstock.com, p. 8; Gado Images/Alamy Stock Photo, p. 9; INTERFOTO/Alamy Stock Photo, p. 10; World History Archive/Alamy Stock Photo, p. 11; Kateryna Kon/Shutterstock.com, pp. 12-13; Vladnik/Shutterstock.com, p. 14; Courtesy National Gallery of Art, Washington DC, p. 15; AP Photo, p. 16; AP Photo/Max Desfor, p. 17; Roman Nerud/Shutterstock.com, p. 18; ProStockStudio/Shutterstock.com, p. 19; JOKE_PHATRAPONG/Shutterstock.com, p. 20.

Cover image: Kateryna Kon/Shutterstock.com.